A Journey of Self Love

(losing 60 Kilograms along the way without dieting or exercise)

By Cheri Ann Revill

Front Cover photo by Rebecca Cook

DEDICATION

Thank you Mum for always believing in Me.

CONTENTS

WONDER

Do you ever wonder about

What if?

What if I...

What if I could...

What if I could be...

Is it possible? Maybe...

What if I could be... Really?

YES I can

I can be anything I choose to be!

By Cheri Ann Revill

PRELUDE

This physical experience is a miraculous wonder of tumultuous emotions, thoughts and experiences. With the beliefs, points of views and judgments of this world, through the beings who create their truths to be the blueprints of not only their life but it seems everyone else who chooses to believe them! Can Life be that simple?

Do we create everything in our life, the good, the bad and the ugly?

If so, why do we choose to keep doing what clearly does not work?

The hardship, the mayhem, the emotional roller coaster of everyday life!

From the relationships we have with ourselves, our parents, our children, siblings, friends and our choice of partners?

Why would we put ourselves through this heartache of trying to please others instead of ourselves?

Where clearly if we were happy others around us

could be happy too and if they are not is that not their issue?

If the choice of feeling good takes the same amount of energy as it does to feel sad, angry, hurt, depressed or pained, would you not choose to feel happy, joy, love and gratitude?

If life could be easy would you not choose for it to be so?

I think people have forgotten how to be happy, not sure how to feel content, or at peace with themselves and life in general.

There are so many influences from others on how to feel, how to live your life, that in most cases there is a state of confusion in exactly what to do!

The question one would ask then is how do I have that, how do I have a life filled with love, happiness, peace, joy and contentment? What is that for me?

These are the sorts of questions I found myself asking when clearly the life I was living was not working for me.

My body would also agree, as my state of health was going downhill rapidly, yet I was too blind to see it until my world came crashing down around me and everything I knew was no longer!

So I had to start again from scratch and try a new approach to life. Looking at myself differently, my body, my relationships with everyone I knew and what worked for me!

This can be a strange concept, as change is not a comfortable feeling for most and they would rather keep going on with the way their lives are rather than be happy, because it was familiar or comfortable.

I have had people say what about your children think of them, and I would say I am!

Would you rather have a mother that was happy, kind and patient, instead of angry, sad and screaming at their children every day?

When are you going to live your life?

Would you wait until your children had left home? When you have retired?

By then it may be too late. Tomorrow could be too late! It only takes a minute for your life to change and then what will you do?

The question that is asked by many is why are we here? What are we supposed to do with our lives? What is the meaning of all this?

For me the answer is, to be Happy!

To enjoy this life, this human experience.

I am grateful for the world we live in right now, with all the luxuries we have, electricity, gas, the technology, the transport that is available, the housing (if we choose to live in one), the choice of where to live, schools, medical facilities, food, clean water, hot water, clothing and so much more!

The choices that we have are phenomenal and all we have to decide is, what, where, when and how! Yes, the choice of what you would like to do with your life is really up to you and how much you believe in your self.

If you believe that you can do anything, anything is possible! If you believe that you have a limited capacity in learning then that is what you will have.

Believe that you can change the world and you will, start with changing how you view your self!

You are an amazing being all you have to do is believe that you can.

ENERGY

Energy is a force to be reckoned with

It can change & shift all beliefs

Everyone & everything has energy running through
them

Energy can vibrate both high & low

We can change what we believe

We can change how we are

We can change how we look

We can change just about anything thus far

All we have to do is make that choice

Believe that we can do

Change how we think

1

and all our dreams will come true

Energy is that powerful

So if you have that much energy

What are you going to do?

By Cheri Ann Revill

MY STORY

Our bodies are a fascinating creation and we are learning more about the human body every day. A number of years ago I was classed as Obese weighing in at 136 kilograms. I had not weighed myself for quite a while, nor had I looked at myself in a full-length mirror. When the scale at a shopping centre showed this number I was completely floored and asked the question how did this happen?

From there I went on a liver cleansing diet and lost 10 kilograms and fell pregnant! Now this was a bit of a shock as it had been 12 years since I had my last child and it took some getting used too. So after a move interstate, (as my husband was with the Defence Force -Army) and the birth of my daughter, losing weight was the last thing on my mind.

I went back to school after returning to Queensland and number 4 child was born.

That year I turned 40, now you are probably wondering whether I tried to lose the weight over the years and the answer is yes. I wasn't always a big girl and I struggled to lose the weight that I had gained after the death of my father and the second pregnancy.

I tried many different diets, that I couldn't even name them all now! Joined gym's, did numerous exercise classes, walked, swam, tried tirelessly and I would lose maybe a couple of kilo's! In the end I gave up.

In 2011, I enrolled into the University of Queensland to do a Bachelor of Health Science Degree. I had been doing this same degree at a college for the past 3 years, which would get me nowhere, I found out.

I had to start again, my youngest son was 8months old, I was at university full time and there were seven at home to look after. By the end of that year needless to say I was a wreck! My marriage had been going down hill for some time, but I thought it would get better if I hung in there and kept trying.

My husband and eldest son had been suffering from depression on and off for a number of years (and apparently so had I, but who has time for that!).

Suffice to say we separated in January of 2012, temporarily at first, to see if counseling helped and after 6 months it was evident that it wasn't, so the separation stayed.

Now I have been doing many self help courses, read books, counseling, meditation courses etc. for 20 years to help with the daily routine of life, children and my relationship.

Some helped for a period of time and others not so much!

Whilst I was separated it occurred to me that I wasn't happy, I was actually miserable and quite stressed, I had psoriasis for many years, which is a physical symptom of stress and I was extremely overweight.

I asked two questions; What is Happiness to me?

What would it take for me to be Happy?

This was quite a revelation you understand because since I can remember I have always done everything for everyone else!

As a child it was whatever it took to keep my Dad

happy and I wanted him to be proud of me.

It wasn't to say I didn't play up, because I did! Hence the reason behind joining the military at 17!

Then I became pregnant within 12 months of leaving home, we were married because I thought it was the right thing to do when you become pregnant (this is what I was led to believe growing up!).

The years that followed, I was told often that I was too young to handle the responsibility of a family and I would not be a good mother and wife. Then when Dad died, I really became lost as I had joined the Army under his influence and I never really liked being a soldier.

The question was asked; Why am I in the Army?

Having 2 young children with both parents in the Defence Force was not such a good idea so I discharged and thought what now?

Money was short as it was for most people, whilst moving around the country following my husbands career and looking after the children, work had to be found. It didn't matter what kind of job as long as money was coming in!Even after deciding to go back to school, it was for me but not for me, if that makes any sense! It was to prove to others as well as myself that I was still smart enough to get a degree.

You see I had lost myself, maybe I had never been found because my life was made up of other people's points of view and judgments of what I should be doing and how I should do it!

I decided, I just wanted to be Happy, I had no idea what that looked like for me. I started to look at everything in my life differently and started to do work on me from within.

I did many alternative therapies, energy work, saw Kinesiologists, studied the Law of Attraction, Meditation and Quantum physics.

I did this every day! I used the tools from everything I had learnt and read or I asked for help if I needed a hand.

During this journey I found that most people are not Happy with their lives and their bodies. I learnt for myself, through trial and error as to what worked for me. For what worked for others didn't always work for me, so I kept trying.

What would I like my life to look like?

What was Happiness for me?

What is love for me?

Learning what Love meant to me was very interesting! How do I project this on to myself, self-love?

I learnt to listen to my body and what my body required as we are all different and we all have different needs. I changed my thought patterns, my points of view and learnt to have no judgments!

Yes that is a challenge as we are bought up on the very foundation to have points of view and judgments about everything!

Now funny enough, over time and I mean over a period of months, I started to lose weight, I never weighed myself but the dress sizes changed. The other changes in the physical sense were I had suffered from migraines for years. Some were to the extent that I had to be hospitalised and drugged with morphine to get rid of the pain. Now headaches are rare, let alone a migraine!

Then there was the skin condition, psoriasis that also plagued my hands and feet for the past six years! That too also disappeared!

I had tried numerous treatments for psoriasis from Chinese herbal medicines, ointments, creams, antibiotics and steroid cream, to UV light, all to no avail!

I used to think I handled stress pretty well obviously not! As the psoriasis was a physical symptom that my body could no longer handle the amount of stress it was under.

By listening to my body, learning to slow down both physically and mentally, learn how to relax, the psoriasis disappeared.

Feelings from within about how I felt about myself changed, I became more confidant in who I was and learnt to like my body and me as a person! As this was happening, I was being pulled in different directions, being told I should be a healer and go back to study more. I started to listen to the opinions of others on which direction my life should be going. I started to lose sight of why I started this journey.

I was living in an apartment building In Ipswich Queensland and my two little people and I would go down to the pool most days.

On this particular day something went wrong and I couldn't tell you why, it just did. I found myself reviving my youngest son, hoping and praying he would come back to me... and yes he did. I am very happy and grateful that he has completely recovered and I had the skills to help bring him back from the brink of death. After this incident it solidified the importance of being Happy.

If I am Happy, my children are happy and life can be so much easier.

I started my own business called Happiness with Ease, I wanted to share and inspire others to create a life of Happiness. Learn and remember how to love self and show others how remarkable their bodies are!

I have lost over 60 kilograms, without dieting and exercising, reduced the stress within my body and I am looking younger!

Throughout this book I will be talking about what I have learnt, the tools I used and how to use them. I hope you enjoy reading this book as much as I have had writing it and that it may help you to remember how to be happy, to love yourself, your body and life can be a little easier than it may have been in the past.

LOVE

Love is in the mind

Love is in the soul

Love is in your heart

Love is all to show

Love is yours to give

Love shows that you care

Love is for you

Love is everywhere

Love is your true gift

The gift of Love is there!

By Cheri Ann Revill

SELF LOVE

Love, the entanglement of Love and all that brings. The meaning of Love creates confusion and chaos in the minds of those who are unsure of who they are and what love means to them. The essence of Love is what creates any relationship, to blossom into something magical or it may become volatile depending on their interpretation of love.

Ideally at the start of any new relationship it could be made quite clear what love means to the particular parties. Show or vebalise their language of love and have it not be assumed that the other person in the relationship has the same version of love as they do!

That being said, with most relationships between parents and children, it is known that they are loved to some degree (though I do realise that may not always be the case).

The language of love is what each individual requires to feel and know they are loved.

There are many differences of how we show love to each other, either through, quality time spent with the person in question, the gift of giving, or spoken in words, affection through hugs and kisses and it could be two or three of these languages together!

Love seems to bring a whole new world, a new insight into the person or people we are loving, the green-eyed monster, jealousy rears its head where it has not even cracked an eyelid before.

The things we do to keep our partner happy, behaviours change, trust comes under scrutiny and even the most easy going person can become stressed, trying to prove their love within the relationship.

What about your happiness and love for yourself?

Let me ask the question... is it not the person themselves that have these issues?

The person that has a certain belief structure, that if you say you love me, you have to love me the way I expect to be loved or that is the end of the relationship?

Then there is the marriage vow until death do you part!

Would you stay in a relationship that is soaked in

misery and hatred until one of you dies?

In my experience your happiness, your self-love is more important and easier to accomplish, than by trying to do so for another.

The same goes for the other person if they were to do the same and then you both come together, both happy with them selves and their lives. Full of self love, confidence of knowing who they are, that the union would not only be easier, would it not flourish, more than one could ever imagine?

The possibilities of a relationship full of unconditional love towards them selves as well as their partner would only strengthen the conviction of each other! I wonder?

Love is quite important in the grand scheme of things, if we don't have love... especially love for ourselves what do we have that is important in our lives.

What does love mean to you? What is love?

This question can stump most people, as we all have a different meaning of what it is to ourselves.

The thing is in my experience, I really had no idea of

what it was, when getting down to the nitty gritty of what Love meant to me.

Don't get me wrong I had a perception of what love was and what I thought love was coming from another, and yet it depended on who was showing that Love!

If it was coming from your parents, your children, spouse, friend... all different!

How do you show love to you?

It is different for everyone, how do you choose what works for you? How do you show yourself love?

As I was going through all the self-help materials that I had acquired over the years, I found that love seemed to be based on a number of things, being grateful for you, stop the judgment and be in allowance of your self.

Honour and Trust your self and then learn to be Vulnerable. This bought up more questions than answers...

What do they mean to me? How do they fall into the category of self-love? How do I show myself this love? So I broke it down and went through each one to find the meaning for me and how do I show it to myself.

Being grateful for you and your body! What a foreign concept!

In my experience, how could I be grateful for me when I didn't even like me or my body? Therefore I started looking at something else. What was I grateful for in my life? My children, they were healthy and whole.

Start off with something small, to be grateful for; a bed, the sun, water simple things, things that we take for granted every day. Now look at your body, you could be grateful that you can read this book, that you have arms and hands to be able to write, hold the television remote, cook, anything really.

Every day find one thing that you are grateful for and then something about your body, each day I did this I found it easier and found more parts of my body I was grateful for. Then I started on me, what was I grateful for about me. I am grateful that I can raise my family.

I can teach my children how to read, write, and ride a bike.

I can learn new things, help others, when I set my mind to it, I found I could be grateful for many things about me! It's a great place to start to find what to be grateful for about yourself. Now you start to believe in you!

We are our own worst critic, I had to learn to stop being so harsh on myself, stop judging me!

I am doing the very best that I can with what I know right now!

A great affirmation to use daily;

'You are doing the very best that you can, with the knowledge that you have on any given subject at that point in time!'

Most of the beliefs, and points of view that we have are from others. These we have picked up since we were children, from our parents, grandparents, teachers, friends, throughout our whole life!

These can be about anything, from how we view the world, to how we view our bodies.

It is your choice you can choose what to believe in, what you believe in creates your life, your body.

There is no wrong or right, just different perceptions, especially when it comes to you and your body.

I decided that I would choose to see me as a beautiful, smart, fun loving, kind, compassionate, generous woman and it no longer mattered what others thought or said about me, I choose to believe in me!

This was something I had to work on a daily, as I had to change my thought patterns.

Once you make that conscious decision you can change your subconscious thoughts too!

I did it and so can you, believe in you, and be in Allowance of you.

Vulnerability is a tricky one and it took me a while to understand the meaning for me and how do I show it to myself! For me it was to break down those barriers, and having forgiveness for all that has happened, for all that I have done, the hurt that I caused and the hurt that I have felt within me.

This can be difficult as I found forgiving others (though it took a little time), was a whole lot easier to do than to forgive myself!

It's Ok to put yourself out there, it's Ok to Love others, trust others, be in allowance of others, be grateful and honour them too, just like you would yourself.

It's Ok, to wear your heart on your sleeve!

If others don't like it, or they try to hurt you with words, again that is Ok because those are the people that have their own world of issues to work out.

Most people project onto others, how they are feeling, it's not you! They want you to feel as lousy as they do, so smile and say it is Ok, do not give them your power. It is safe to be loved and to love. I can say this now and it did take a few times before I actually believed it. I had given my power over to others, thinking it was me, it was my fault, but it wasn't.

Other people have their own issues their own demons they are fighting and now I have the confidence, the strength to say that's Ok, I know this is yours not mine.

Honouring yourself, how do you put yourself first when you have been told as soon as you become pregnant that the child comes first, when you get married your husband comes first and foremost?

It is funny because as a child this was not the case, my mother came first, my father would put her first and always said make sure we always bought her a gift for mothers day and her birthday. Always help your mother out and treat Mum with respect!

That belief was not in my own family because it certainly didn't happen to me.

I had to learn to put me first, honour me, that I deserve the time, the money and the help!

The children didn't suffer because of it either as I thought they would. What did happen was everyone became a lot happier because I was happier and then, I was also treated a lot better.

If you love yourself and honour you in the way you deserve others will do the same. You deserve to honour yourself, take some time out for you! Don't wait for someone else to get you the gift you always wanted or the flowers or whatever it is that you wish for.

Start with taking some time out for you once a week, put some money aside until you have enough to get yourself that special something.

I would always be disappointed when my birthday or Christmas came as I seemed to miss out because everyone else was put first and there was never enough money for my special something.

Now I buy my own gifts and I don't wait until it is a special occasion!

Believing in you is to be able to trust yourself. How do you know if you have a trust issue?

If you have trouble trusting others it is something within you that is the issue! You have to be able to trust yourself, rely on your inner knowing. You may have heard it called intuition, gut feeling, when you have that bad feeling you shouldn't do something but you go ahead anyway and it all goes wrong!

Your inner knowing, trust that you know what is good for you. What feels right, it sits well with you and you feel light. If it doesn't feel right, it can make you feel like the world is on your shoulders, you feel heavy, know that feeling?

Trust that, trust yourself, be aware of the world around you, listen to your body and notice the difference within you.

These 5 factors around Love helped me to learn to like, and then love myself, as I had never felt that towards me ever in my life.

Now how do you project love onto your body when you don't like the way you look? It is interesting and it did take a while for me to understand how. I found that, it doesn't matter what size or shape you are if you don't learn to like, then love you now, it won't matter what you do, you will never be happy with your body.

How much weight you lose or how much you try to change how you look, you still won't like what you see! Learn to love you at this present moment with how you look and you will be surprised in how much of an affect it has with helping make those changes.

I started with something I liked about my body, I like the colour blue and the colour of my eyes are blue, so I could say I like my eyes.

Then I went to a part of my body that I didn't like which was my arms.

Then I asked the question why didn't I like my arms and I remembered a time when I heard someone tell someone else that they had tuck shop ladies arms! I took that on board and believed I had that too, so I covered them up all the time! It was someone else's belief and as I started to change that belief my arms were not anywhere near as bad as what I thought they were.

I did the same when it came to my thighs, I had carried most of my weight in my thighs. Though I remember a time when I was a lot thinner and I was doing roller derby, a photo was taken of my thighs and put up on the notice board of the roller skating rink with a note, which labeled them as tree trunks!

Again it was some one else's belief of what they saw,

the thing is when others put parts of your body down it is normally how they feel about their own body.

Nobody can change how you feel about you but you! Change how you see yourself, change your points of views, your judgments, your perceptions of your body and you will never be affected by what others say again!

One of the biggest myths about finding yourself, learning to Love yourself is that it is a lonely journey.

Now it may feel like this at the beginning of discovering who you are, what you like to do, to be, but as you learn more about you, you will find that you enjoy your own company!

Look forward to some alone time, then you will find the things that you love to do, read a good book, watch the sunset/sunrise, go out for coffee, or going out for a drink. It may be just to sit and take in the beauty that is around you, go for a walk anything really.

The journey to self-discovery can also show you, how to love you and your body.

There was a video taken of a forensic artist drawing portraits of just random people, there was a screen put up between the person and the artist, then they had to describe them selves for the artist.

Then another person who had seen this same person had to sit down and describe them for another portrait. Consequently there were two completely different pictures.

How we see ourselves is definitely not how others see us! When we are describing how we look to someone else, it is completely different to how others see us.

'If you could only see the beauty within you, the way that I see you!'

This is so true and as we learn to Love ourselves we can start to see how truly beautiful we really are!

YOU

You are Amazing

You are Unique

You are Beautiful

You are Sleek

You are Wonderful

You are Unbeatable

You are Happiness

You are Incredible

You are Unforgettable

You are Lovely

You are Awesome

You are a Superhero

You are all these things and MORE...

Love being the best of YOU!

By Cheri Ann Revill

Your Body

Our bodies are amazing, you are made from a cell, from that single cell your whole body was created from and it took 9 months to develop and another 5 years to fully form. Those cells keep replicating, they die and make new ones for the rest of your life. Each cell has a powerhouse called the mitochondria and it produces more than enough energy to light up a city block for 3 months!

So times that by the trillions of cells that make up you, think you have more than enough energy?

Going back to the cells replicating themselves, making new ones every day, did you know you actually have a brand new body in less than 7 years? Your body is capable of so much more than you may realise, all you have to do is ask!

There are eleven systems that make up your body, The skeletal system (bones), muscular system (muscles), nervous system (brain, spine and nerves), cardiovascular system (heart and blood vessels), lymphatic system (lymph nodes and vessels, immune system), respiratory system (lungs), digestive system

(stomach, liver and intestines), urinary system
(bladder, kidneys and urinary tract), reproductive
system (female or male reproductive organs),
endocrine system (consists mainly of hormonal
glands) and the integumentary system (hair, nails and
skin).

Now all of these systems play a role in the total
function of your body but for me the most important is
the nervous system, it has control over your whole
body. If the nerves do not connect to each organ they
don't work, if the spine is not connected to your brain
the body doesn't work and how you think and feel
affects how your body functions overall. Everything
you think, feel and do affects how your body works on
a daily basis. What you eat, how much you eat, how
much your body moves, how you are feeling, all has
an effect in how your body looks and functions.

Your whole existence depends on your respiratory
system working as well. We are unable to live if we
cannot breathe! Are we breathing properly, so the
body is receiving enough oxygen for every organ in
the body? Most of us do not use the full capacity of
our lungs when we breathe especially the lower lobes

which effects how much oxygen transference there is into the blood.

The deeper and longer we breathe the more oxygen goes into the blood stream, which is then pumped, to every area of our body. This also helps with the healing process and helping our bodies work at optimal capacity.

The digestive system is also very important with the healing process and in helping your bodywork at optimal level. The body receives its nutrients through the intestines, so it is important that the walls of the intestines are healthy enough for them to absorb what the body requires.

The performance of your body is dependent on the amount of vitamins, minerals and oxygen that it actually receives via the blood stream and how well it travels through out your body.

Are we not responsible for not only what we eat, drink and the amount of movement we do, but also how we think and feel? Everything is tied up into one package, if we feel good, are aware of our thoughts, listen to our bodies and what it requires in the way of food, fluid, movement and relaxation.

It would change our whole body makeup and what is possible when it comes to our health, how we age and our overall well being.

Listening to your body is a new approach for most. Your body will tell you everything you need to know, what to eat and how much to eat.

This is quite important because your body requires certain elements to function. Your body needs to be working in unison, for it to be able to heal itself and sometimes during this process it will need a helping hand.

Everyone's needs will be different that is why what will work for one will not work for another. By listening to your body you will receive exactly what your body requires! I have found muscle testing your body to be extremely effective. I do this for everything concerning my body. I needed more Good oil (Omega 3s) for the function of my digestive system also to eat less red meat.

My immune system required more antioxidants. This can be found in berries, capsicum or you can also find it in liquid form called Mangosteen.

My skin required avocados and khale. These are only some of the foods, I have had, to help heal my body over the last couple of years, but they may not be what your body needs. Less alcohol, sugar and coffee, very little fast food and I found over time the urge to have these things will became less and less. I started to feel good and have more energy and confidence to do things I loved to do. I also found I was eating a lot less as my body had said that is enough.

If you are present when you eat, take the time to enjoy your food; don't eat it on the run.

Whilst you are eating, you will notice that the taste of your food will change, this is your body's way of saying it has had enough. If throughout the day you feel hunger, ask your body, 'Are you hungry or are you thirsty?'

Most bodies don't have enough water, which is really important as your body is made up of 70% of water. Taking time out for yourself, rest and relaxation is also something your body requires to help with the healing process. Sleep, your body also needs to have enough sleep for it to function effectively the next day.

Muscle testing can be in different forms, a Kinesiologist uses your arm, by asking your body questions and how your arm reacts through the muscles moving.

What I did was to stand straight, feet together, hands by my side and asked a question. Go on you try it! Stand up, stand straight, feet together, hands by your side, now lets find out what is yes and no for you. Your body will either move backwards or forwards to yes or no so we have to find out which is which for you.

Ask a question that you know the answer is YES, like your name... Body is your name...? Did you move? Did you move forwards or backwards? Now it could have been the slightest movement, you have to be a little patient, your body is not used to you asking it anything!

Lets try a NO question, you could ask the question of even someone else's name or if you just eaten, Body are you hungry? (See how I snuck that in... we will get to that a little later!) Now you should know which way yes is, for me it is forwards and No for me is backwards.

There will be times where your body will rock from side to side, that means you need to ask a different question. Maybe even a more specific question.

This will take some practice, I did this everyday more than once and I asked my body everything. I now don't have to rock backwards and forwards, which is a relief to my children as they thought I was a crazy lady and especially my teenagers, who would not come shopping with me!

Now dieting, not a great word and did you feel how your body reacted to that word? It's not a great word as it has Die in it! In saying that, there may be a particular diet that does work for your body for a period of time.

You will know as it is easy to stick to and it makes you feel good! Your body requires all different kinds of food, I know all about the food pyramid, the medicinal purposes of food (onions and garlic in food helps with colds and flus).

This was really interesting for me because I had to retrain the way I thought about food, to what my body required and actually listen to my body.

There are times when your body may only want something in particular and if you go out and order a meal it may only want one thing on the plate! The key is to know what your body would like to eat and how much it would like to eat. You don't have to eat everything that is on your plate, as most of us have been trained to do!

At home you can muscle test yourself but if you go out, you may not want to be rocking all over the place.

There is a trick, it will be the first thing you think of, or the first thing you see either on the menu or in the cabinet!

Yes the first thing, don't have an argument with yourself, Trust Self. Yes; trust your intuition. With most things in your life go with the first thought it always turns out to be the right one! Going back to food, you are now sitting down to eat, be present with your food, enjoy it, make the noise, (yes I know you know what I mean).

Now that you are being present notice how the food tastes, as you are eating. As you are eating notice when the taste changes, it becomes bland!

Yes that's when your body is telling you it has had enough!

In my experience it has worked for me and it became easier the more often I did it. Please don't get upset with yourself if you forget or you feel it's not working. Keep trying don't give up, and see what happens.

It could be the smallest thing you may notice that gives you the encouragement to keep going!

You may feel happier, less stressed as it takes away all the decisions you have to make about what to eat.

Then see or feel the difference not only on the out side but also within you.

I know I did!

Movement sounds and feels so much better than exercise, which is derived from the word exorcism! Say both words and feel how your body reacts to each word. Interesting huh? Your body loves to move, find what it loves to move to!

It could be going for a walk, somewhere you love to go to; a park, bushwalking, the beach, even in your backyard if you love going outside to have some peace and quiet.

It could be you love to dance, put on favourite tune and dance around the house. It could be roller skating, riding a bike, going for a swim, any kind of movement that makes you feel good and it doesn't feel like a chore. Some people love going to the gym, going to aerobics, doing yoga or pilates, lifting weights.

The point is that you are excited to do it and it brings a smile to your face. That is when you know that your body loves it and enjoys that movement. See you have started to listen to your body.

JOY

The simple things bring such joy

Everyday things, we see all the time

Some you may not even see, it could be a sense of
smell,

touch, taste and things that you may hear

What if we could stop for a while and sense the joy
that life can bring

The sound of children's laughter or the pitter-patter of
rain on a tin roof

The smell of fresh bread or fresh ground coffee in the
morning

The touch from a loved one or the soft touch of a
feather

The taste of cool clean water on a hot day or
snowflakes melting on your tongue

There are so many different things all around

Every individual has their own special joy filled
moments

That makes life every day an incredible joyous day.

By Cheri Ann Revill

Thoughts and Feelings

Quantum Physics - How does it work?

Your thoughts and feelings have become hardwired into your brain so it becomes second nature. It is so automatic it is in your subconscious, you think it as soon as you get up, you listen to it through the media, read about it in magazines etc. it is everywhere. Your thoughts create, how you feel. How?

The thoughts you have create an electric current which runs through the neuron pathways within your brain to the nerve endings called synapses.

The current is then sent to another part of your brain called the Hypothalamus.

The Hypothalamus then creates the chemical that produces your feelings, called peptides. So if you feel sad, the hypothalamus makes that peptide for that feeling, which is then sent to the cell receptors (they surround every cell) like a key into a lock and there you have that feeling. Same goes for happiness, anger, love, any feeling, and a peptide is created and sent to the cells to coincide with that thought pattern!

These pathways are set over time, but they can be changed! Change your thoughts, change how you feel and believe it. Then a different thought pattern has occurred! How about an example?

Think of someone or something you love. Notice how your body reacts to this feeling, you feel warm and tingly inside and it brings a smile to your face. Now think of something or someone you find challenging. How does your body feel now? Your body reacts to your thoughts, which creates your feelings within your body!

To change thought patterns it takes time, you have had these thoughts for years and it will take a conscious effort on a daily basis to change them.

You can change how you think, it is possible to make the decision and create a different and better thought pattern for you. In my experience it worked for me, it took many months to change how I thought about myself but it was worth it! I have lost 60 kilograms in 12 months without dieting and exercise, I feel and look better then I have ever in my life!

Everyday we are bombarded with how we are supposed to look, supposed to feel, our susceptibility to disease, how we age, what happens to our bodies after having children, after we turn 30, 40, 50, 60 it's all down hill from here! I choose to believe in something completely different, who made up these rules?

My body is capable of healing itself with some help from both alternative medicine and scientific medicine from time to time. I choose to be Healthy and I can say I have not had as much as a cold in 18 months.

If my body requires help with either antibiotics or other alternatives, I'll give my body every opportunity to help heal itself.

This is where listening to your body comes into play which I explained earlier in the book. There have been so many stories where people have cured themselves from disease, been able to walk again, see again and so much more, all because they choose to believe differently than what they were told! How is this possible?

Your mind, your thoughts create your beliefs, which create your life and your body.

Most of you would have heard about meditation and visualisation, some find this quite a challenge. In another chapter I go through a meditation, which is quick and easy, I have a life and children, when would I find the time to sit for hours and meditate?

Visualisation does mean to picture what you would like to happen but that is not so easy for some, though if you think it and believe it, it is! Yes same principle applies, if you sit or lie down and think about what you would like your body to be or do it will have the same affect.

You can strengthen your immune system, strengthen your bones, your nervous system, anything really!

Think of rushing water going through all of your systems and as it is flowing through them you may find there are blockages along the way.

These can be disintegrated with ease until the water is flowing easily through your whole body and down into the earth. Do this to your energetic field as well, which surrounds every living thing on this planet.

You may notice the difference when you come across someone who is unhappy. You may feel drained and unhappy within yourself after leaving their presence. When someone is happy and excited you can feel the difference it makes to how you feel as well!

When you walk into a room, after someone has had an argument, that saying 'you can cut the air with a knife!'

That is their energy field giving off what they are feeling on the inside, you can clean and clear that as well. Then think of a colour you love and feel that flowing in and around your entire body, your body will feel so much better.

From there anything is possible believe in your body and the capabilities that is has and you may be surprised!

What does the Law of Attraction have to do with our bodies?

Life is full of possibilities and extraordinary chances. All you have to do is choose, decide and grab the opportunity with both hands and run with it! Have the belief, the faith and the conviction that it will work out and work out way better than you could ever imagine! Life has many of these but most do not take them, as fear takes over or change doesn't suit them, as it is too uncomfortable.

Most people like to have control over every area in their lives, but do they really have that control? Control is an illusion, no one has control over most parts of their lives. What will be will be, you do the best that you can do, think the best thoughts and feelings you have, on any given situation. The rest is left up to the Universe, all you can do is wait and see what happens.

How you think and feel decides the outcomes of all situations, all aspects of your life.

There is a vibration you give off through how you are feeling. This vibration can be low or high, this is your energy field that surrounds you and it attracts others that have a similar vibration. Everything on this planet gives off a certain amount of energy, like attracts like!

The Law of Attraction is what they call it! This goes with everything within the life that you live. Especially when it comes to your body, how you think and feel about your body, about you comes about. Everything you have heard, read, seen in this lifetime with anything to do with your body, that you truly believe, happens!

It may be conscious thought or it may go much deeper than that as we are bombarded with so much information.

Whether it is true or false is irrelevant, it is what the individual believes to be true that comes to fruition! You create your life, you create and generate everything that happens to you in your life, the good, the bad and the ugly! The more you are convinced that only great things will happen that is what you will create in your life, relationships, money, and health all depends on how you think and feel about these things!

If you believe you are financially abundant, you feel it and think it, have the conviction within your whole being, it will happen.

Now it may not happen when you think it will happen or how you think it will happen, but it will!! Believe in you, believe in the power of you and you can create the most amazing life ever!

Do things you never thought possible, see the most amazing things, have the happiness you deserve, Love like you have never loved before and be extremely grateful for all that you have and all that you have become and all the you will be!

Love, happiness and gratitude are the highest frequency vibrations there are and if you feel these with every cell of your being there is no holding you back, you will fly, you will soar, you can conquer the world, if you so desire.

Anything is possible!

Have you ever heard someone say if they eat a particular food it will go straight to their thighs or their bottoms, and does it? So if you change your belief in your body, if you believe that you are beautiful, trim, lean, have clean and clear skin, soft silky hair, listen to your body's needs and the possibilities are endless!

You see I had to accept all that has happened in my life, I created my life. Consciously and subconsciously, one way or another I created it!

The feelings (vibrations) that we have about everything we don't want, will attract that which we don't want and the feelings we have about what we do want attracts back, what we do want.

The Law Attraction doesn't establish the difference it just knows how much feeling you project out, on any given subject.

If it takes the same amount of energy, which would you choose?

Do you remember anytime in your life where you have said I really don't want…. and what happened? Did it come about? Think about it!

Believe

Believe in you

Believe in what you know

Believe in the power within you

Don't be afraid to let it show

For if others see it come from you

Then maybe it is possible for them too

The only way to change the world

Is to start with the belief in you!

By Cheri Ann Revill

Believe

How many of us have a burning desire within our soul bursting at the seams to come out? Follow our desires, our dreams, knowing what that dream is and taking action on it!

Never giving up! Keep going, have faith, believe, know that it will come true, it will eventuate in the very near future.

No matter what obstacles may come up, or how many hiccups that life may throw at you, you handle them with the greatest of ease knowing it won't stop you moving forward, making your dream a reality.

Though for some, their Dream has been lost or forgotten. Find your fire, your dream, your greatest desires in life, believe you can make it come true, know you deserve it and do whatever it takes for you to make that dream come true!

You have the Magic within you, the power, the will the determination, the love and the belief you can do it! You can do anything, be anything and have anything, if you believe in yourself!

Go forth and show the world what you are made of, what gift you can give them, because we all have a gift to share with everyone.

We are all amazing beings and our greatest gift is to share our Love with each other.

No Matter what you have done, where you live, what size, shape or how old you are it is never too late start! All you have to do is make that decision, make that commitment, you are worthy of being the best possible you. Take one day at a time, and you can turn your life, your body, your health, your happiness into the best decision you ever made. It may take months, years for you to be where you would like to be, it all has to do with the journey.

The journey takes you along the path to happiness, to a healthy body, a positive mind. As you start to change, others will start to notice, what have you done? You look amazing, you look happy!

How did you do it? They see you and you give them hope! Yes it is possible. As I started to change and lose weight, I went and visited a girlfriend, we have been friends for over 20yrs. She was amazed by the transformation and started to ask questions and you could see the possibility that maybe she could do it too!

It's the planting of the seed of hope that gives the thought that maybe just maybe I can do it too.

My friend did start, she is doing it one day at a time, going on her journey and one day I know she will get to a place where she is happy and also has self love for herself. I know because she said to me 'if you can do it, I can do it too!' That's all you need, to spread that seed of Hope that anything is possible, all you have to do is believe in yourself and then others will too! That is my hope with this book, by writing about my journey, my experiences on what I learnt, that I might be able to give all of you hope!

You can do anything, be anything, have anything all you have to do is Believe in yourself, I know I believe in you!

Many of us feel that we will like ourselves once we are certain shape, a certain size, dye or change our hair style, etc., but once we have achieved our aim, how we feel on the inside has not changed. Start changing how you feel about you, how you look now! Change your belief system about your body completely. You have been listening to everyone's points of view on how your body should look, since you were little.

Your friends, family, television, magazines, newspapers, all suggesting your body should look certain way, and it is all your fault that you look the way you do!

This is not the case, you are already beautiful, perfect, as you were born that way!

You are a miracle you were created from a single cell, these cells keep replicating for the rest of your life, and how they replicate is up to you!

Start with something small, what do you like about your body? What do you like about you?

Then you can add to that, every day.

Then look at what you don't like, why don't you like it?

Where did that come from?

Something you have heard or seen?

Is it really your point of view?

Most of our points of views and beliefs have been derived from others since the day we were born.

You will look like someone in the family due to your genetic structure!

You should look like this or this will happen to your body when you get to this age.

You should be this height and weight!

Once you are married or have children this will happen to you! This is not completely true and a way for you to know this is how it sits with you. Some of these beliefs will not feel right and some will. That is your intuition at work and many have lost this over the years or have not been taught how to use it. Like your gut feeling, you just know something, don't know why but you just do!

This is your body telling you what is true for you.

Everyone is unique, you are not supposed to be or do or even look like everyone else! You are you, be proud of you, how you look and you are capable of so much more than you are led to believe. All you need to do is have the belief, the faith that you can do it, your beautiful regardless of what anyone else says.

I was extremely lucky as a child that my parents told me that I could be or do anything I wanted to be and so it never occurred to me that I couldn't until I was an adult and then others told me differently.

I was told that due to my weight that I wasn't a good mother, wife, unable to find a certain type of work, but looking back those people started telling me those things before I even started putting on weight!

When people have a point of view about you, it is normally their own issues they are dealing with because they have been judged on that exact same thing. Let them believe what they want to believe, let them have their opinions of you, of themselves.

Believe in yourself, you can do it, you can love yourself for who you are! In my experience once I learned to like myself again and then love all of me, that is when things started to really change. I could look at myself in the mirror and say hello beautiful, thank you body you are amazing! I allowed my body to look how it would like to look and by listening to my body I was able to lose weight and look younger!

Breathe

How many of you actually sit down for five minutes and breathe? Relax, de-stress, and take a time out? Who has time for that right? Breathing is one of the easiest forms of meditation that you can do and you don't have to do it for hours to receive the benefits from it.

Most people don't receive enough oxygen intake into their bodies, which improves the bodies healing capabilities and functionality.

When we breathe we don't use all of our lung capacity and the key is to get as much oxygen down into the bottom lobes of our lung so that the transference of oxygen into the blood stream is at optimal level.

If there is more oxygen in our blood, then our organs will receive more oxygen so they will be able to function better and heal quicker! So lets give it a try now, shall we?

Ok; take a deep breath, actually take 3 deep breaths! Now as you take the next breath see if you can count in your head how long you inhale (breathe in) for and how long you exhale (breathe out) for. Breathe in 2, 3, 4 Breathe out 2, 3, 4 Breath in 2, 3, 4 Breath out 2, 3, 4.

Can you feel the difference within your self, your body is more relaxed, you have stopped thinking (which is a good thing!) and I can feel a smile forming on your face!

The key is to do this a few times a day but increase the count. On the first day just get used to setting aside 5 minutes to breathe, no matter where you are, in the car, at the office, even before you go to sleep which can help clear away the stress of the day to help you go to sleep. I can now count up to 9 while breathing in and10 while breathing out.

Oh yes, I nearly forgot, it is just as important to breathe out a little more than you have taken in to get rid of as much carbon dioxide as you can. The more oxygen that is left in your body the better!

This breathing meditation will help you relax, as we seem to hold all our stress in our bodies. It can be seen in the lines on our face or appear on our skin, in the form of excma and psoriasis.

Stress is one of the reasons our bodies don't function at an optimal level. It forces us to rest and recuperate, when we don't listen to it. Pain is normally our body screaming at us, trying to tell us something is wrong and it is the only way we will listen to it.

BEAUTY

Beauty is here

Beauty is there

Beauty is everywhere

Beauty is shared

Beauty is hidden

Beauty is sensed

Beauty can not be ridden

For Beauty is everlasting

A treasure to behold

Beauty can be seen in anything you hold

Beauty can be in the smallest of places

Beauty can be seen in the most magnificent of faces

Beauty is found no matter where you look

Beauty can even be found in any kind of book

Beauty is found even within you

All you have to do is Believe

There is Beauty in YOU!

By Cheri Ann Revill

Anything is Possible

Starting each day anew, the rainfalls down blanketing the earth washing away all that was. The smell of the rain is fresh and new, the glistening of the raindrops on the grass, the leaves, the flowers tell a new story. Everything is beautiful, lush and green after a good fall of rain.

We enjoy the after affects, the earth cools down, we cool down, the animals cool down everything gets a drink and everything blossoms after a good downpour.

As this happens upon the earth how can we relate this to our inner being?

How can we create this analogy to our everyday living to make us as human beings Happier?

The analogy can be used either when we are swimming or in the shower as we are going through the water or having the water flow over our human form feel it wash away the past. Feel it wash away everything that was and we can start anew. Isn't that a beautiful feeling?

What could you do if you had the opportunity to start over, start again, with no belief's, no judgments of ourselves, no points of view on how we see ourselves and the surrounding world we live in!

What would you do? What would you like to have in your life that you thought was not possible? What would you like to be, do or have that you didn't have before?

So you wake up one morning and you have the chance to have a do over.... I mean don't forget what once was, it shaped you to who you are now.

Be grateful for those experiences, the lessons, the love, the friendships and all that has happened to you right up to this point.

Now what would you like your life to look like now if you could choose anything? If you could choose anything, would it be a house, a car, to travel, clothes, anything that you thought would make your life better? Or would you choose to be happy?

Would you choose to have amazing people in your life, that don't judge you and loved you for who you are, unconditionally?

Would you choose love? You project how you feel about yourself to others around you, they see how you feel about yourself, how you treat yourself and then do the same, treat you the same way.

Could you love you unconditionally? What is Love to you is probably a better question to ask. Most people do not know what love is to them, they think it is based on actions from others, a feeling of either lust or jealousy. Would you love yourself that way, the way you love your partner now, your family, and your friends?

How do you love you unconditionally?

Self love, believing in your self where do you start if you have never believed in yourself before.

Loved yourself, not even liked you?

Where do you start?

You start from the beginning.

You start from a place where is believable for you.

What part of you do you like? What are you good at?

It could be writing, love for books, being outdoors,

being around other people, family, find something you like to do and do more of that. Is there something about your body you like, eyes, shape of them colour, size?

Ears, nose, eyelashes, eyebrows, skin, lips, teeth, hair, fingers, fingernails, find something you like about your self and that is where you start from.

How you see yourself is not how others see you. This seems to be a challenge for most when it comes to finding something about themselves they like, and then adding to it. That is the thing, trying to add to it every day or the one thing that you would like to change into something you love!

For me it was my eyes, the colour of my eyes, then my lips, I liked the shape of my lips and their natural colour.

I liked my ears because of the way they were shaped and I loved having them pierced.

From there you can add to your list of what you like about your self. Have you found something that you are good at? Do you have a Dream? Something you have always wanted to do? Or something you love doing already but think you are not good enough at it so decided to let it go?

Go back and think about how it made you feel, did you feel good, excited looked forward to doing it?

That is what you should be doing! When you are doing something that brings joy it changes how you feel, how you think, how you see the world and your life!

Do more of what you love and see how it changes everything! When you feel comfortable with looking at something you don't like, ask yourself why do I not like this part of myself, my body? I found that the parts of my body I didn't like, were not as bad as I thought they were, nowhere near it!

As I became more comfortable with myself, I stopped covering them up. Then I went to the next part of my body and worked on how I felt about it. The thing is, it is your thought patterns that have to change, which does take time as they are ingrained over years of looking into the mirror and judging your self. You probably don't even realise that you are thinking that way any more, as it has become second nature, it is set in your subconscious.

You need to be aware of your thoughts, making a conscious decision, by changing the words you use about yourself.

I hate my body, I don't like how the skin hangs from my arms, or the stretch marks on my thighs, the cellulite on my hips and so on. Where did you hear that any part of your body was wrong for being that way? Family, friends, media?

Everyone has something they don't like about themselves and they will always tell everyone about it and then the others they are talking to, will also take it onboard!

There in lies how thought patterns are created. The thing is everyone has a point of view on something, if it doesn't feel right to you don't take it on board, they are their issues not yours!

Once you start to look at yourself differently and realise what you see is not what everyone else sees, change your thinking and how you feel about your self will change too!

This process is done over time and you have to work at it every day. If you have one of those days when you don't feel like changing your thought process or forget to do it that is ok! Start again tomorrow!

There is no right or wrong, you do the best that you can do, with each day, there is a new start.

Be gentle with you, don't judge you, we are our own harshest critic, so go easy and it will get easier as time goes on "the more you do it the easier it gets'. You are breaking a habit, like smoking, drinking, it is something you have to work at everyday until it becomes second nature.

Hello beautiful you are looking amazing today lets go out and show the world how awesome you look today! If you believe in yourself others will believe in you! It is not only your body, it is with anything in your life, changing your thinking to a more positive thought pattern.

Then you will find everything will change. Change words like wrong to right, can't to can, ugly to beautiful. You would be amazed at the difference a word can make to change how you are feeling.

There will be days, I am not saying there won't be that you will feel uninspired, under the weather and so forth. New day, new beginning, new start! What makes you happy? What brings a smile to your face? What brings that feeling of excitement to your body?

Think about that, do that and it will help lift your mood to a happier one. You have to find what makes you feel good, it is a matter of remembering that feeling.

You might have to go back a few years, but there will be a time when you have felt good, find a happy memory!

Then when you have found it you can go back to that memory time an again, you start to feel good, bringing a smile to your face and sit with it for a while.

Then look around you and see other things that you like, that make you feel good.

Go outside and sit in the sun, look at the butterflies, bugs, grass, blue sky, anything really, things in your home that make you feel good! Finding the things that make you feel good is a great start to helping you feel good within.

Your Happiness is within you, you just have to remember what it is or go and find what makes you happy. Your thoughts and feelings are all connected, that is why sometimes it is a good idea to try not to think! I know that is easier said then done, distracting your self with something that makes you feel good is a great idea.

Gratitude! We can all be grateful for many things we have in our lives but are we truly grateful for the mundane every day things we take for granted?

Like running water in our homes, that water which we can drink and cook with.

The electricity and gas that is provided to our home that gives us hot water!

The electricity that provides the light, the warmth and to cook the food we eat.

A refrigerator to keep food cold so it doesn't go off! Television, not only the electricity that helps it work but the receiving of a signal so that we may be able to watch it.

Beds to sleep on, pillows for comfort and blankets, to keep us warm. Clothes to wear for protection and warmth, shoes also provide the same benefit.

A roof over our heads to provide protection, heaters, fans, chairs, tables, couches, washing machines, cars, petrol, roads, etc. the list goes on and on and on!

Then there is not only yourself but also your family, your children, providing comforts for them, so that they are protected, kept warm or cool, hydrated and bellies full!

Money no matter in what form, or where it comes from, how much as long as it is something to help provide the every day necessities so that we may survive in this world!

Are we truly grateful for what we have in our lives? There are so many that go without every day needs that most take for granted. How long would we survive if we went without a few of these things?

I am Happy and Grateful for all that I have, for all that

I am and for all that I will be!

I am truly grateful that I have the basic needs and that I can provide them for my children.

The thing is we can say we are grateful but when it actually happens, to go without any of our daily needs, that is when you are truly grateful for what you have!

Until then it is just words without the feeling of gratitude, for the hot water to bathe in, the heating to keep you warm, a fridge/freezer to keep your food in, warm clothes, shoes, clean water, food in general or a roof over your head to protect your children from the elements.

When you have to live without even one of these things or more you are then placed in a situation of being grateful for it, when it does return.

Love is also something we take for granted either from out parents, children, friends, partner ... do we acknowledge their love or do we let them know that we Love them and we are grateful for them being a part of our lives?

One day may be too late! Letting the ones we Love know how we feel about them regularly can give us peace of mind. That if anything was to happen, they know that they were loved and were appreciated!

Life is full of different experiences and we can choose the life we lead.

Remember to be grateful for everything in this life, not just the big things but the little ones too, the everyday ones, the mundane ones, because you never know when you may have to live without them!

NEW DAY

With the light of a new day

Brings the smell of crisp clean air

There is dew from the night air on the ground

and birds in flight singing with flare.

The sound of the animals greeting one another

The whistle of the wind through the leaves in the trees

To the kiss of sunlight on the flowers all around,

What an amazement array the new day brings.

The start of any new day

Brings a new perspective on life

We can start this day anew

A clean slate, wiped clean, no past in sight

So I choose to start this day

With a fresh new perspective

I choose to live life to the fullest

That is what I am going to choose!

By Cheri Ann Revill

ABOUT THE AUTHOR

Cheri Ann Revill Author (A Journey of Self Love), Public Speaker, Innergetic Coach and CEO of Happiness with Ease
Mother of four children and Grandmother, lives in New South Wales, Australia.
On a Journey to find Happiness after a life once known crumbled after 23 years.

www.ingramcontent.com/pod-product-compliance
Lightning Source LLC
Chambersburg PA
CBHW070555290526
45790CB00002B/692